PROPOLIS

Nature's Most Powerful Infection Fighter

Terry Lemerond

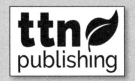

The purpose of this book is to educate. It is not intended to serve as a replacement for professional medical advice. Any use of the information in this book is at the reader's discretion. This book is sold with the understanding that neither the publisher nor the authors have any liability or responsibility for any injury caused or alleged to be caused directly or indirectly by the information contained in this book. While every effort has been made to ensure its accuracy, the book's contents should not be construed as medical advice. To obtain medical advice on your individual health needs, please consult a qualified health care practitioner.

Copyright © 2023 TTN Publishing, LLC, Green Bay, WI

All rights reserved. Except as permitted under the United States Copyright Act of 1976, no part of this publication in any format, electronic or physical, may be reproduced or distributed in any form or by any means, or stored in a database or retrieval system without the prior written permission of the publisher.

Library of Congress Cataloging-in-Publication Data is on file with the Library of Congress.

ISBN: 978-1-952507-47-2

Interior: Gary A. Rosenberg • www.thebookcouple.com
Editor: Kathleen Barnes • www.takechargebooks.com

Printed in the United States of America

10   9   8   7   6   5   4   3   2   1

Contents

Chapter 1. Meet the Beehive's Immune System, 1

Chapter 2. What Bee Glue Means for Humans, 6

Chapter 3. Vanquish All Kinds of Viruses, 10

Chapter 4. Banish Bacteria, Too, 15

Chapter 5. Eject All Those Other Stubborn Nasty Bugs, 22

Chapter 6. Prevent and Treat Cancer, 26

Chapter 7. And there's more…, 35

Chapter 8. What You Need to Know, 40

Chapter 9. Doc to Doc, 43

References, 49

Index, 53

About the Author, 57

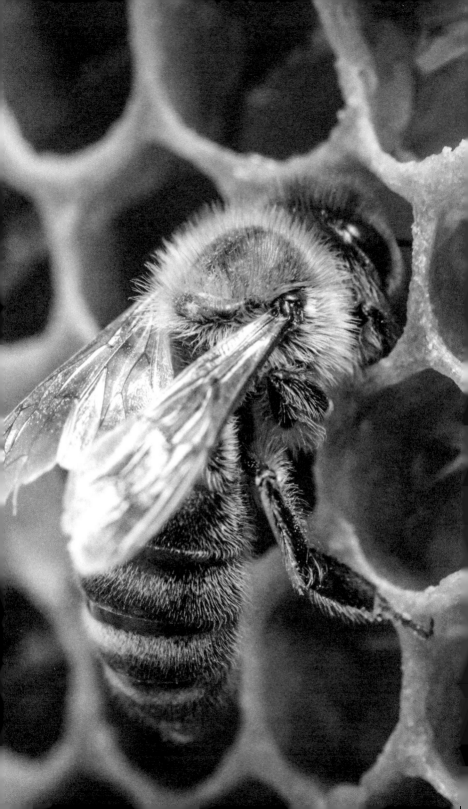

CHAPTER 1

Meet the Beehive's Immune System

Blessed bees!
 Bees are responsible for dozens, hundreds, maybe even thousands of functions in our ecosystem that guarantee our food supply.

Albert Einstein has often been famously misquoted as saying, "If the bee disappears from the surface of the earth, man would have no more than four years to live. No more bees, no more pollination, no more plants, no more animals, no more man."

While it's now generally agreed that Einstein probably never made this statement, it is known that he had a deep interest in biodiversity, so the apocalyptic prediction contains at least a kernel of truth.

Pollination

Honeybees are primary pollinators, which means their ceaseless buzzing from flower to flower supports our entire food chain. Bees are responsible for pollination of 85% of human food crops. In fact, according to the World Wildlife Fund, one of every three bites of food we consume is dependent on pollinators, including honeybees.

They also make essential contributions to the pollination of feed crops for animals and wild crops that sustain trees and other plants, birds and wild animals that are the foundation of the complex network that is our entire ecosystem. Bees and their pollination services ensure the continuity of food sources for all humans and animals by creating seeds for next year's crops. They're also essential to the pollination of cotton and flax crops that clothe us.

Humans have been cultivating honeybee colonies for at least 20,000 years. Our far distant ancestors had at least some idea of how important they are to the web of life.

Honey

How sweet it is! Of course, only honeybees can produce honey. Honey has a host of health benefits, including prevention of cancer, heart disease, gastrointestinal diseases and diabetes. It's also known to increase athletic performance and heal wounds, and even treat eye infections.

So where does propolis come in?

Propolis is the protector of the entire bee colony. Its name reflects its reason for being: pro—from the Latin "for" and polis, "the city." "For the city" is exactly what Propolis does. Stay with me.

Can we take a moment here to navigate the complex world of a beehive?

A beehive is like a city with about 50,000 members, maintained year-round at a temperature of about 50 degrees Fahrenheit and 90% humidity. Honey is the hive's food. To keep the temperatures warm enough in winter, the bees cluster together and exercise their flight wings. They subsist on honey in the cold and scarce times. To accomplish this in cold climates, the colony must consume about two pounds of honey a week.

Propolis is a brown, sticky, waxy resin produced only by honeybees by mixing resins from leaf buds and tree sap flows with their saliva and beeswax. The bees load these sticky resins into the pollen baskets on their hind legs and carry them back to the hive. Sometimes called "bee glue," honeybees use propolis to repair and seal openings, damage, and cracks in their hives. Just like fixing the problem you might have with a drafty house in winter, bees would not survive winters without propolis.

It's also used to seal the cells in the honeycomb where the larvae grow to keep them safe and to ensure the future of the colony.

Propolis also has two other important functions:

It keeps the colony safe by forming barriers to keep out external enemies like snakes, mice and lizards. In fact, if a predator manages to make its way into the hive, the worker bees immediately kill it and effectively mummify it with propolis so a body that is too heavy to remove is prevented from contaminating the hive.

And here's where we bring out the brass band—TA-DA! Propolis keeps the hive healthy by blocking all types of disease- and infection-causing microorganisms that would be expected to thrive in that 50-degree, high humidity environment.

Let me repeat that because it's so important:

Propolis keeps the hive healthy by blocking all types of disease- and infection-causing microbes that would be expected to thrive in that 50-degree, high humidity environment.

In fact, beehives are scientifically validated as among the cleanest environments in the natural world, all because propolis protects them and prevents disease with a powerful barrier that wipes out bacteria, fungi and viruses.

Propolis is the colony's immune system. It's easy to see how the bees' natural defense substance could be of benefit to humankind. But we're getting ahead of ourselves.

Let's take a closer look at what is in propolis:

Researchers have identified more than 300 elements in propolis, most of them nutrients called polyphenols, a class of antioxidants.

What's an antioxidant? It's any nutrient that prevents cells from oxidizing, a process of cellular decline that promotes disease and speeds aging. Antioxidants are essential for disease prevention.

Going further down the scientific rabbit hole, those polyphenols in propolis come largely from a category known at flavonoids, produced as part of a plant's immune system and passed on by bees when they collect pollen and resin, and form propolis.

These potent compounds give propolis its ability to overcome invasion by viruses, bacteria and fungi.

And it's an excellent source of the anti-inflammatory compound called caffeic acid phenethyl ester.

Plus, propolis is a rich source of vitamins, minerals, enzymes and essential oils.

Even though the leaf and tree sap sources for propolis may vary for honeybee colonies around the world, researchers find that colonies everywhere are protected by its impressive pathogen-fighting properties.

WHAT YOU NEED TO KNOW

- Propolis is a sticky, waxy resin produced by bees to protect their colonies.

- In nature, propolis helps seal the hive against predators and weather, but most important, it maintains the colony's health and security in a high-risk environment of high humidity and warm temperature.

- Propolis has been scientifically validated as a potent antimicrobial, which means it can eliminate viruses, fungi and bacteria.

CHAPTER 2

What Bee Glue Means for Humans

Propolis has profound implications for humans, ones that have been validated by science for decades.

Maybe the first chapter of this book gave you a clue about the way the beehive's immune system can help and even protect humans at this challenging time in human history.

It's important to recognize that the conditions in a beehive—high humidity, and warm temperatures are quite similar to the human body's climate.

I'm talking about its nearly unparalleled antimicrobial properties. With the prevalence of rogue viruses in our world today, what could possibly be more important than a way to conquer viruses, bacteria, fungi and other dangerous pathogens naturally and effectively?

Propolis is an incredibly complex molecule with hundreds of components. Its healing power comes mainly from phenolic compounds, like flavonoids (including quercetin, galangin, chrysin) and derivatives of hydroxycinnamic acids (caffeic acid, cinnamic acid, p-coumaric acid). Propolis also contains other healing molecules, including aromatic aldehydes, diterpenes, sesquiterpenes, esters, lignans, alcohols, amino acids, fatty acids, vitamins and minerals.

We'll be going into that in detail in the coming chapters.

A brief history

The medicinal properties of propolis have been recognized since ancient times. It was particularly recognized in the Arab cultures and it is even mentioned in the Koran. It's been used for an astonishing variety of purposes ranging from toothpaste to mummification.

I know. Mummification is interesting. If you're not squeamish, think about the bees' use of propolis to "mummify" intruders in the hive so their bodies would not decompose and cause infection in the colony. There is evidence propolis was used by ancient Egyptians as early as 5500 BC. Propolis was carried into war by Roman soldiers as early as 100 BC for its wound healing properties, as a tonic and face and body cream as well as to address a range of feminine health issues.

The ancient Jews called propolis "tzori" and its medicinal uses are extolled throughout the Old Testament. Even Hippocrates was known to use propolis for wound healing internally and externally.

In 1600, propolis was listed as an official drug in the London Pharmacopeias.

Russian soldiers carried propolis, sometimes called "Russian penicillin," into the battlefields of World Wars I and II.

When antibiotics were discovered slightly less than 100 years ago, science turned away from those ancient remedies, but in today's world of rampant viruses, pandemics, antibiotic-resistant bacteria, and fungal infections that claim as many as 25 million lives around the world every year, those vital medicinals have reclaimed their rightful place in disease treatment.

A treasure beyond measure

Propolis is a classic combination of nature *and* nurture. It surely is a vital link in the survival of bees and their contributions to pollination and the human food chain, *plus* its healing properties that quite literally save human lives.

Of course, in this time of rampant microbial attacks on humans, a natural substance that conquers viruses and harmful bacteria is a treasure. One that does all of this without the need for expensive laboratory tests and without side effects or a buildup of resistant microbes is a treasure beyond measure. We'll learn more about this in Chapter 3.

Beyond the natural antibiotic properties of propolis, propolis has long served humankind by helping heal wounds, even those that were severely infected. We'll explore this further in Chapter 4.

We're going to dive deeper into the lesser-known benefits of "bee glue" and its invaluable contributions to human health.

It wipes out fungal and parasitic infections, making it a broad spectrum antimicrobial unparalleled in the world of natural healing, as we'll explore in Chapter 5.

It is a powerful medicine against chronic allergies, as we'll see in Chapter 6.

And, I'm pretty sure you've not heard about the powerful anticancer properties of propolis, but you'll get all the information you need to avail yourself of this powerful tool for healing in Chapter 7.

Then there is a plethora of ailments against which propolis is a proven healer, including:

- *H. pylori* bacterial infections that cause gastric ulcers
- Burns

- Periodontal disease
- Tooth decay
- Vaginitis
- Acne
- *And more*

What's the common ground? Of course, they are all infections caused by harmful bacteria. We'll learn more about the power of propolis to banish bad bacteria in Chapter 8.

Thanks for joining me on this quest to learn the secrets of the bees' gift to humanity.

WHAT YOU NEED TO KNOW

- Propolis has been a recognized healing medicine since ancient times.
- It is a proven antiviral, capable of eradicating today's most rampant viral infections.
- Its antibacterial powers have been proven to heal the medical world's most challenging infections, including *Staphylococcus aureus*.
- It helps conquer chronic allergies.
- It prevents and treats a wide range of cancers.
- It's proven effective against fungal and parasitic infections.

CHAPTER 3

Vanquish All Kinds of Viruses

Viruses are the scourge of today's life no matter where on Earth you live.

Since the pandemic changed all of our lives in March of 2020, it has presented challenges we never would have imagined. Many of us have contracted the coronavirus that causes Covid-19. Some have debilitating long-term effects. Sadly, some of us have lost loved ones.

The peaks and valleys of contagion continue and are likely to have a profound impact on our lives for years, perhaps decades to come.

Propolis provides a promising answer to Covid-19 and the host of other viruses, including flu and colds, that plague humankind.

In fact, in just a short time, there has been credible published research on propolis as an effective method for treating and preventing Covid-19.

Propolis has long been recognized as a powerful natural antiviral treatment. Remember the bees and their use of propolis to keep all sorts of infections out of their hives and to clean them up, creating an almost sterile environment if pathogens were able to enter the hive? Well, propolis can do the same for the human organism as well.

Bees are vulnerable to a wide range of diseases, including at least 22 identified viruses.

Of course, humans are susceptible to many more viruses. We have all experienced the multitude of viruses that cause colds and flu at one time or another. We've touched on the SARS-CoV-2 viral infection that causes the dreaded Covid. We'll go into that in detail in a page or two.

But, how often do we think of other viral infections that have had such a profound impact? How about HIV, the virus that causes AIDS? Or the HPV (human papillomavirus), a sexually transmitted disease that can result in several genital cancers? Or the viruses that cause hepatitis, Ebola and dengue fever that periodically reach epidemic and even pandemic levels in scattered parts of the world?

Propolis has been studied and found to be safe and effective against all of them.

The Brazilian researchers who published a comprehensive review of published studies on the antiviral effects of propolis in early 2021 enthusiastically conclude that propolis works better than antiviral drugs that diminish their own effectiveness by triggering viral mutations and variations. Propolis has no known side effects, as opposed to antiviral drugs like acyclovir, interferon-a and oseltamivir, that can cause kidney injury, neurological damage and more.

It all starts with innate immunity—the human body's natural immune system that fights off microbial invaders of all types.

The human body is amazingly equipped to fight off pathogens. When innate immunity fails to stop a viral infection, the adaptive immune response kicks in recognizing a virus it has seen before, like a flu virus you experienced two years ago.

Propolis has been labelled an "immunomodulatory" substance, meaning that it can turn up the volume on the immune response when needed.

When any part of the immune system unleashes its lethal weapon to destroy disease-causing microbes, including viruses, damaging inflammation can occur. This can include potentially fatal lung damage caused by influenza viruses, which take over half a million lives a year worldwide.

Propolis was shown to stop the growth of the H1N1, H0N1 and H3N2 viruses as well as "retroviruses" like HIV and a similar virus that cause a form of leukemia and the polio virus.

Another plus: Propolis helped heal cold sores caused by a herpes simplex virus quickly.

Propolis and Covid-19

Obviously, SARS-CoV-2, has only been known to science since early 2020. Information about and understanding of this terrible disease is constantly evolving, as is the virus itself and its numerous variants.

Yet, as of this writing in mid-2021, there have been several credible and important studies on the effectiveness of propolis against the virus that causes Covid-19.

SARS-CoV-2 is part of a large family of coronaviruses that includes the common cold. These coronaviruses usually cause upper respiratory tract illnesses. It differs from other coronaviruses because it is highly contagious (some variants are even more contagious) and the symptoms can be devastating, even deadly, as we all know.

Most of us have probably heard about the "cytokine storm"

that can cause multi-organ failure, frequently resulting in death, not only in Covid patients, but in people suffering from a variety of other viruses.

Solid laboratory, animal and human research confirms the immunomodulatory effects of propolis by boosting the fighting power of both the innate and adaptive immune systems, plus it helps strengthen antibodies, works as an anti-inflammatory, thus sidestepping the inflammatory side effects that can cause cytokine storms.

Propolis, administered in combination with Covid vaccines, resulted in the body's ability to produce more antibodies and, therefore, better immunity to future challenges and evolving variants.

It's a case of nature nurturing humans by providing propolis, a natural healing substance.

In a study published in the journal *Biomedicine Pharmacotherapy*, a consortium of Brazilian and US researchers concluded, "Propolis has also shown promise as an aid in the treatment of various of the comorbidities that are particularly dangerous in Covid-19 patients, including respiratory diseases, hypertension, diabetes, and cancer. Given the current emergency caused by the Covid-19 pandemic and limited therapeutic options, propolis is presented as a promising and relevant therapeutic option that is safe, easy to administer orally and is readily available as a natural supplement and functional food."

Safety

Propolis has been proven safer than antiviral pharmaceutical drugs, without any serious side effects, even in pregnant women and people with diabetes. It has also been shown to protect the heart, lungs, liver, kidneys and other organs. Some researchers have suggested that propolis might enhance the effectiveness of antiviral drugs currently being used to treat Covid. Plus, it did not result in an interaction with prescription drugs that a patient might be using or other antiviral therapies like those frequently used by people with HIV.

WHAT YOU NEED TO KNOW

Propolis has long been scientifically validated as an effective and safe antiviral remedy. Research shows its effectiveness against:

- SARS-CoV-2, the virus that causes Covid
- Colds and flu
- HIV, the virus that cause AIDS
- HPV (human papillomavirus), a sexually transmitted virus that can cause cancer
- Herpes viruses
- *And many more*

It works by strengthening the immune system by increasing the production of antibodies against the viruses and reducing inflammation.

CHAPTER 4

Banish Bacteria, Too

Bacteria are smarter than humans, by a long shot. That's how they have been able to get a foothold (if they had feet!) into a wide range of human diseases and disabilities and evade humankind's smartest efforts to overcome them.

Scientists and beekeepers have long known that bees are prone to bacterial infections. It probably won't surprise you to learn that propolis, which helps keeps the hive safe from disease, also helps prevent and cure bacterial infections as well as in humans.

This protection ranges from a simple infected cut that got infected because you didn't keep it clean enough to serious food poisoning caused by the *E. coli* bacteria that you might have picked up at a family picnic, to potentially life-threatening infections like largely hospital-originated infections caused by the *Staphylococcus aureus (MRSA) bacteria.*

There's more. One study even confirms propolis' effectiveness in fighting over 600 types of bacterial infections!

Researchers have credited propolis with "broad spectrum" antibiotic properties that "enhanced the safety of conventional antibiotics." There's even some research that suggests propolis might even enhance the healing properties of pharmaceutical antibiotics.

Science is still catching up with traditional healing, so more research will undoubtedly reap even more ways propolis promotes healing.

It's those magical polyphenol compounds called flavonoids that are responsible for most of that special protection the propolis provides. In some cases, the flavonoids simply enhance the immune system and, in others, they act directly on the bacteria causing an infection.

Artepillin C, one of those flavonoids, has been found to kill the staph bacteria that causes potentially deadly infections.

Another extract of propolis called kaempferide is confirmed against a variety of skin infections as well as the *Staphylococcus Saprophyticus, Enterococcus Faecalis and Listeria monocytogenes* bacteria that cause urinary tract infections, abdominal infections, meningitis, cellulitis, encephalitis, miscarriages, vaginal infections and more. All these nasty bacteria are notoriously antibiotic resistant.

I could go on with a whole alphabet soup of the types of bacteria that propolis has been proven to combat, but you get the idea. This is serious stuff and propolis is serious medicine.

Antibiotic resistance

Numerous studies have indicated that propolis has no toxicity and no side effects in animal models or humans.

You surely don't remember the time before antibiotics were "discovered," but the idea that pneumonia was quite literally a death sentence 100 years ago may surprise you. Deaths from tuberculosis, cholera and typhoid fever were common. In fact, strep throat and even simple ear infections that spread to the brain took a deadly toll before the days of antibiotics.

The discovery of penicillin by British scientist Sir Alexander Fleming in 1928 changed all of that and saved countless lives. Just one example: The survival rate for people who contracted bacterial pneumonia dramatically increased from 20% to 85% between 1937 and 1964.

Antibiotics are estimated to have saved 200,000 lives every year and added as many as ten years to life expectancy in the first few decades after Sir Fleming's discovery of the "miracle" drug.

I started this chapter noting that bacteria are smarter than humans. Here's why: Bacteria have an uncanny ability to evolve (mutate) at a breathtakingly rapid pace, resisting all efforts to kill them.

Yet, almost from the beginning, antibiotic resistant strains of disease-causing bacteria emerged. Initially, this growing antibiotic resistance led to the evolution of the original penicillin and other antibiotics, and the addition of numerous other antibiotic drugs like amoxicillin, doxycycline, tetracycline, sulfa drugs, mycins (E-mycin, Biaxin, Zithromax) and floxacins (Cipro, Levaquin).

Now, those drugs are significantly less effective against common bacteria. They are killing us again. Those smart little buggers have developed the ability to defeat the drugs that were designed to kill them. Not only are these disease-causing bacteria not killed by the miracle drugs, they continue to grow. Infections caused by antibiotic-resistant bacteria can be difficult or even impossible to treat.

More than 2.8 million antibiotic-resistant infections occur in the United States each year, and more than 35,000 people die as a result, according to the Centers for Disease Control and Prevention (CDC).

Sadly, pharmaceutical companies have lost interest in developing new antibiotics to combat the wild proliferation of antibiotic-resistant bacteria, leading to a new worldwide crisis of deadly infections.

The World Health Organization warns, "Without urgent action, we are heading for a post-antibiotic era, in which common infections and minor injuries can once again kill."

Causes of antibiotic resistance

Scientists are now in general agreement that antibiotic resistance is caused by human ignorance.

1. **Overuse:** Antibiotics are only effective against bacterial infections. They have no effect on viral infections like colds and flu. In those early decades, doctors were so enamored by the new drugs that they indiscriminately gave them to everyone who showed up in their offices with a sniffle. This led to rapid evolution of the bacterial strains that quickly learned how to overcome the standard antibiotics. Today, many patients demand antibiotics even though they will be ineffective.

2. **Inappropriate use:** Antibiotics have an amazing quality of helping people feel better fast, so they fail to complete the entire course of treatment designed to eradicate the infectious bacteria.

3. **Farming:** The widespread use of antibiotics to prevent infections and stimulate growth used for meat, dairy and fish farming that leave antibiotic residues in foods we consume, leading to antibiotic buildup in our bodies and increased antibiotic resistance.

4. **Poor infection control in health care settings:** This is largely due to the inappropriate use of antibiotics and inadequate hygiene among health care workers. Hospitals are increasingly becoming overwhelmed with the numbers of patients with all types of infections, making infection control more difficult.

5. **Poor hygiene and sanitation:** We would hope the pandemic has taught us about handwashing and social distancing to prevent spread of viral and bacterial infections, but perhaps not. Hygiene in food preparation and storage, poor water quality and demand for meat and fish products raised using antibiotics have all increased antibiotic resistance in communities.

6. **Lack of new antibiotics:** The development of new antibiotics has fallen to an all-time low. Bacteria resistant to the current pharmacopeia are winning the race, to our peril. Without new antibiotics, we are running out of options for treatment.

Propolis gives us hope

Propolis offers hope and, yes, even excitement. Not only has propolis been proven effective against a wide range of bacterial infections, it doesn't create antibiotic resistance (because it isn't an antibiotic in the pharmaceutical sense). There are some cases in which propolis can enhance the effectiveness of pharmaceutical antibiotics against resistant bacteria.

Crucial 2018 study results confirmed that propolis is effective against the *Staphylococcus aureus* that causes potentially deadly MRSA. Better yet, repeated use of propolis in a lab setting did not result in any resistance.

Other US research confirmed the effectiveness of propolis against *Escherichia coli* and there is evidence it is effective against *Mycobacterium tuberculosis,* the bacteria that cause tuberculosis, a disease that is on the rise worldwide.

Here is just a partial list of bacteria that are proven to respond positively to propolis treatment:

Gram-positive bacteria

Bacillus cereus, Bacillus mesentericus, Corynebacterium spp., Corynebacterium diphtheriae, Diplococcus pneumonae, Enterococcus spp., Mycobacteria sp., Mycobacterium tuberculosis, Staphylococcus aureus, Streptococcus: critecus epidermis faecalis mutans, pyogenes, viridans, sobrinus, Micrococcus luteus

Gram-negative bacteria

Branhamella catarrhalis, E. coli, Helicobacter pylori, Klebsiella ozaemae, Klesbsiella pneumonae, Proteus vulgaris, Pseudomonas aeruginosa, Salmonella: choleraesuis, dublin, enteritidis, exneri, gallinarum, pullorum, typhimurium, paratyphi-A, paratyphi-B, typhi Shigella: dysenteriae, sonnei

Maybe the bacteria aren't as smart as humans? Or as smart as Mother Nature?

WHAT YOU NEED TO KNOW

- Propolis protects beehives from all sorts of infections, including bacterial infections. It has the same effect on humans.

- The discovery of antibiotics was a double-edged sword: It saved millions of lives threatened by bacterial infections and it led to the development of antibiotic super strains of antibiotic-resistant bacteria.

- Propolis has been scientifically validated as effective against a wide range of bacterial infections, including many that are antibiotic resistant.

CHAPTER 5

Eject All Those Other Stubborn Nasty Bugs

I'm sure that the preceding chapters have made you a fan of propolis. I sure am! In fact, I think it belongs in every household's medicine cabinet and first aid kit.

But there's even more. While viruses and bacteria may be the best known of harmful microbes, they are not the only ones.

Combination infections

Before we get to other pathogens like fungal and parasitic infections, I want to bring up diseases that can be caused by a combination of microbes. Ear infections (otitis media) is a common childhood malady that can be caused by a virus, bacteria or both.

If you're a parent, most likely your child has had an ear infection, since five out of six children has had at least one ear infection by the time they are three years old. It's not surprising that ear infections are the number one reason children are brought to the doctor.

Ear infections stem from an obstruction of the eustachian tube, the canal that connects the middle ear with the throat and equalizes the pressure between the outer ear and the middle ear. When that canal gets blocked by a viral or bacterial infection or both or even an allergy (think of a sore throat, sniffles or a cough), fluid backs up into the ear.

Childhood ear infections are becoming more and more difficult to treat in an era of increasing antibiotic resistance.

Propolis provides worried parents with an answer. Clinical studies have shown that propolis can reduce the duration and severity of ear infection, reduce the need for antibiotics and prevent recurring infections. By activating the immune system and the natural defense system, propolis offers safe treatment and prevention without the use of synthetic drugs that can have serious side effects.

The ability to treat infections that may be caused by a combination of pathogens is part of the beauty of propolis: You don't need to know the exact pathogen that causes an illness. Think of propolis as a broad-spectrum way to knock out the bad guys.

Fungi

The *Candida* yeast family, especially *Candida albicans* (a fungus), can be the cause of a great deal of discomfort in the gut, the mouth and the genitourinary system. This is largely because the overuse of antibiotics (the name quite literally translates to anti-life, meaning they wipe out almost all gut bacteria, friendly or not) opens the way for yeast overgrowth in various places, primarily in the gastrointestinal tract.

It's not surprising that, like antibiotic resistance, there is antifungal resistance. It's not surprising that resistance has developed to the fluconazole, the primary antifungal drug widely used to treat candida overgrowth.

Turkish research confirms that propolis is effective against a broad variety of candida infections, including those resistant to pharmaceutical drug treatment, and Brazilian research confirmed it is especially effective against thrush, a common yeast infection of the mouth, particularly in people who wear dentures.

Another Brazilian study showed propolis is an effective treatment for vulvovaginal candidiasis, more commonly known as vaginitis, also caused by yeast overgrowth.

Parasites

Nobody likes to think about it, but parasites are fairly common causes of a number of human maladies.

Giardia, caused by contaminated water and a variety of parasitic worms, caused by inadequate food and personal hygiene, are the most common in children and adults. Blood-sucking parasites like ticks, mosquitoes, fleas and lice can also be a source of disease.

Malaria, caused by the *Plasmodium* parasite, is not common in the US, but the cause of 400,000 deaths worldwide every year, is one of the mostly deadly parasitic diseases.

Again, propolis provides hope and perhaps even a solid answer to parasitic infections.

Iranian lab and animal research confirms that propolis is an effective treatment for malaria, and Indian research confirms that finding and the effectiveness of propolis for a variety of parasitic diseases in humans and animals including giardia (from fecal contaminated surfaces, especially water), trichomoniasis (sexually transmitted), toxoplasmosis (from cat feces or contaminated meat), Chaga's disease and leishmaniasis (tropical diseases transmitted by insects).

This is further confirmation that propolis offers a simple, effective and far-reaching solution to a broad range of infectious diseases.

WHAT YOU NEED TO KNOW

The bottom line: You don't need to know whether an infection is viral, bacterial, fungal, parasitic or has a combination of causes. Propolis has been scientifically proven to be effective against a broad range of infectious diseases.

Among the fungal diseases for which propolis has been tested and found effective:

- Oral thrush
- Vaginitis
- Gastrointestinal upset

Propolis has also been proven effective against the following parasitic diseases:

- Malaria
- Giardia
- Toxoplasmosis
- Trichomoniasis
- Chaga's disease
- Leishmaniasis

Propolis has also been shown to be effective against some drug-resistant forms of treatment for these diseases.

The ability to treat infections that may be caused by a combination of pathogens is part of the beauty of propolis: You don't need to know the exact pathogen that causes an illness. Think of propolis as a broad-spectrum way to knock out the bad guys.

CHAPTER 6

Prevent and Treat Cancer

Cancer is a complex disease that develops in many different ways and requires multiple types of treatment.

Propolis has components that fight cancer in at least five ways (maybe more—new ones are being confirmed frequently!) and has been clinically proven to be effective at slowing, stopping or even eliminating cancer growth in some of the most deadly forms of the disease.

Cancer killed more than 606,000 Americans in 2020, according to the National Cancer Institute (NCI).

The most common types of cancer in the U.S. are (in descending order, according to estimated new cases):

- breast
- lung and bronchial
- prostate
- colorectal
- melanoma
- bladder
- non-Hodgkin's lymphoma
- kidney and renal
- endometrial
- leukemia
- pancreatic
- thyroid
- liver

Remember this list. It will become very important in a few pages.

Let's take a brief look at each of the ways propolis has been scientifically validated for its potent effects against cancer.

About 1.8 million people will be diagnosed with cancer this year. A sobering fact: The NCI says approximately one in three people diagnosed with cancer will die of the disease.

Probably the most impressive review of the research on propolis and cancer comes from a group of scientists at Chulalongkorn University in Bangkok, Thailand who confirmed its anticancer effects against several ways that cancer grows and spreads:

- neutralizing free radical damage
- stopping out-of-control cell lifespans
- optimizing immune system response
- stopping metastasis, cells from spreading throughout the body, usually through the bloodstream

Antioxidant

We need oxygen. Without oxygen, you will die in a few minutes. When you breathe in oxygen, oxygen molecules (oxidants) are normally converted into water by your cells. When this conversion is incomplete, so-called "free radicals" are generated. This can happen for many reasons, including insufficient oxygen to the brain (hypoxia), emotional stress, infections, pollution, and toxic exposure, etc. That results in the disease-causing process called oxidative stress.

Those dangerous free radicals generated through oxidative stress cause cellular damage and dysfunction, resulting in disease.

Cell Deterioration

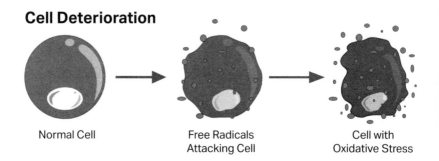

Normal Cell → Free Radicals Attacking Cell → Cell with Oxidative Stress

Normal cells have a built-in antioxidant system, which declines with age and becomes unable to neutralize free radicals. This is the underlying cause of many of the diseases of aging, including cancer, heart disease, diabetes and Alzheimer's.

Propolis is a rich soup of anticancer nutrients, including those flavonoids I mentioned in Chapter 1 and a variety of compounds known as polyphenols that have a blanket antioxidant function.

This explains a part of the anticancer activity, since cellular oxidation is a major factor in almost all human diseases of aging, including cancer. Antioxidants, like the polyphenols in propolis, are well-studied and proven to prevent cancer and treat existing cancers.

Apoptosis

All cells in the human body have a specific life span programmed into our DNA. Our cells are living and dying every single day of our lives and each cell is programmed to adhere to that finite lifespan, a biological process called apoptosis. In a strange sequence, chemical messages are sent to the cells telling them quite literally to commit suicide. The DNA of the cells is destroyed by enzymes released as a result of these chemical messages. The cell's surface bubbles away and chemical sweepers usher the dead cells out of the body, but not before they have reproduced themselves.

Healthy red blood cells live for about four months. They are replaced with new cells that are an exact duplicate of parent cells. White blood cells live for a year or more, but skin cells live only two or three weeks; colon cells die after about only four days. The human body replaces an astonishing one million cells per second.

Sometimes things go wrong for reasons not yet fully understood by modern science, when apoptosis fails and cells don't die at the end of their normal lifespans or they do not reproduce exactly the same as parent cells.

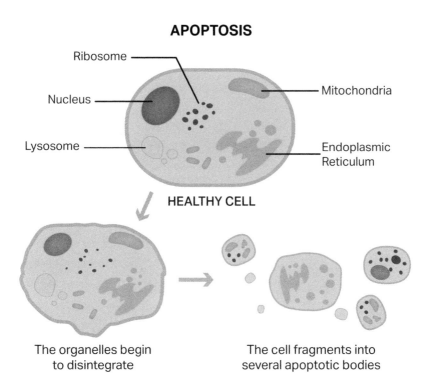

With cancer, those immortal cells can continue indefinitely, clump together to form tumors and may eventually kill the patient.

Recent research confirms that propolis induces apoptosis confirming its effectiveness against several types of cancer, including breast, prostate, colon, pancreatic, brain and oral cancers, leukemia and melanoma, a deadly type of skin cancer.

Propolis re-establishes communication between cells, literally getting the cells' lifespan back on the right track and wipes out tumors.

Immune booster

In earlier chapters, I've already taken a deep look at the impressive immune-boosting qualities of propolis. Of course, these extend to helping the human body fight cancer.

CAPE (caffeic acid phenethyl ester) is one of those powerful polyphenols present in abundance in propolis. It kills rogue cells and regulates inflammation, both major factors in most types of cancer. It also boosts apoptosis.

In the simplest terms, this means that propolis tells the immune system to control abnormal cell growth.

Angiogenesis

All living beings require nutrients in some form to survive. Cancer cells and cancerous tumors are no different.

Angiogenesis is the process of growing a blood vessel network to nourish a cancerous tumor and allowing it to thrive and grow.

It stands to reason that cutting off that blood supply and oxygen, thus eliminating nutrients, will stop a cancerous tumor from growing and spreading.

Numerous studies show that propolis, and especially CAPE, sparks angiogenesis by helping shrink the tumor-feeding network of blood vessels.

In addition to CAPE, other ingredients of propolis such as artepillin C, galangin, kaempferol, and quercetin showed an ability to stop angiogenesis and starve tumors.

Tumor suppression

Cell damage means damaged DNA, so cells are no longer able to reproduce themselves exactly. This results in the formation of tumors, among other problems.

Taiwanese researchers found that propolis stops the cycle of melanoma cancer cell growth. Based on past statistics and the fact that the rate of melanoma has been growing for the past 30 years, the American Cancer Association estimated that over 90,000 Americans were diagnosed with this potentially deadly form of skin cancer in 2018 alone.

Similar results have been seen in studies of pancreatic cancer cells and in glioblastoma cells, an aggressive form of brain cancer. Both of these cancers are notoriously deadly. Pancreatic cancer kills 90% of its victims within five years and glioblastoma kills 96% within five years.

Tumor suppression is credited to essential oils in propolis—like benzoic acid, benzyl alcohol, vanillin, and eugenol—that are confirmed to reduce human colorectal cancer tumors.

Metastasis

Cancers want to hedge their bets. Not only are those cells capable of feeding themselves, they are also capable of entering the bloodstream and lymphatic system and spreading far and wide in the human body, the process called metastasis.

Metastasis is the spread of cancer from its origin, known as the primary cancer site, to another part of the body. While metastasis is not an automatic death sentence, it will become one if it is not stopped.

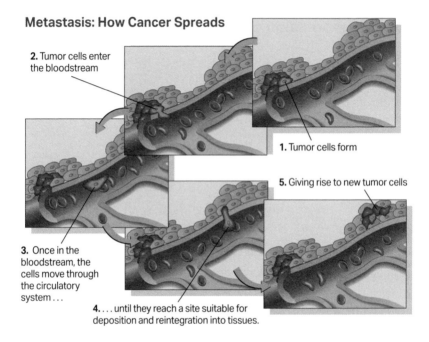

Metastasis: How Cancer Spreads

1. Tumor cells form
2. Tumor cells enter the bloodstream
3. Once in the bloodstream, the cells move through the circulatory system...
4. ...until they reach a site suitable for deposition and reintegration into tissues.
5. Giving rise to new tumor cells

It probably won't surprise you that propolis stops the spread of cancer as well. The metastasis itself and the spread of cancer stem cells explain how cancers can erupt, and be "cured" only to re-emerge, perhaps a few years in the future. That's because those cancer cells can enter the bloodstream, lie dormant and eventually get a foothold in another part of the body. A broad body of research confirms that propolis can stop stem cell migration and metastasis.

In conclusion

Think back to the list of the most common cancers from the beginning of this chapter. I'll repeat it to save you the trouble of paging back to the list.

- breast
- lung and bronchial
- prostate
- colorectal
- melanoma
- bladder
- non-Hodgkin's lymphoma
- kidney and renal
- endometrial
- leukemia
- pancreatic
- thyroid
- liver

Here's what's important:

Propolis has been proven to be an effective treatment and preventive for every single one and then some, like pancreatic cancer and brain cancers that are less common, but extremely deadly.

Among the researchers who have investigated the anti-cancer properties of propolis, there is nearly universal endorsement of propolis as a treatment and as a complementary treatment to conventional cancer treatment. A few even suggest propolis might enhance the effectiveness of conventional chemotherapy treatment. All agree that propolis is safe and effective.

WHAT YOU NEED TO KNOW

Propolis is well-studied and proven to be effective against the most common and the most deadly types of cancer. It works in a broad range of ways to prevent and treat cancer by:

- Boosting the immune system to fight off cancers before they begin
- Stopping wild cell division that forms tumors
- Telling those wild cells to die at the end of their normal lifespan
- Stopping the terrible disease-causing effects of free radical oxygen species
- Enhancing the effectiveness of conventional chemotherapy drugs.
- Stops the spread and re-emergence of cancer

CHAPTER 7

And There's More...

I imagine you are duly impressed by what you've already learned about propolis. I certainly am!

When I first started researching propolis several years ago, I was hoping to find a natural substance that could offer protection against the broad range of microbial infections, including viral, bacterial, fungal and protozoan infections that challenge humankind. I hoped to find a way to help us all heal. I think I have succeeded.

In propolis, I found the answer to microbial infections, and much more than I expected.

As I mentioned in the previous chapters, propolis has been a traditional medicine for millennia. Now many of the benefits of propolis have been scientifically validated, including some you might not have considered.

Here's a brief recap of more impressive powers of propolis:

Diabetes: There's promising research in this area of great health concern. One human study from Iran showed that propolis helps lower blood sugar and other markers for cardiovascular, kidney and liver malfunctions that are of extra concern for people with Type 2 diabetes.

Other Iranian researchers reviewed 14 studies on propolis and found that propolis lowered glycosylated hemoglobin

(HbA1C) levels that indicate blood sugar levels over a period of months, another major preventive for the long-term effects of high blood glucose. The same study also showed strong evidence that propolis helped reduce cholesterol levels. This offers significant protection against cardiovascular disease, for which people with diabetes are particularly vulnerable.

Oral and genital herpes: Propolis is an effective treatment for cold sores, caused by the herpes simplex virus (HSV-1) and genital herpes, caused by the herpes simplex virus 2, HSV-2. Yes, these are caused by the same virus that causes chicken pox, so they are viral. These findings confirm the antiviral powers of propolis.

Propolis is also a safe and effective treatment for shingles, caused by the related herpes zoster virus. One Czech study published in the *German Journal of Pharmaceutical Sciences* showed that propolis was just as effective as acyclovir, the shingles treatment of choice in conventional medicine. Other studies suggest the effect is similar for the herpes simplex viruses.

Allergies: Propolis lowers blood levels of eosinophils, white blood cells that increase the inflammatory response in both allergies and asthma. Allergies are caused by the body's overreaction for a substance that isn't really harmful. It happens when the immune response starts running out of control. Indian research says that propolis not only increases immune response when it is needed, it modulates or lowers the immune response when it is inappropriate, like we see in allergies and asthma.

In what will seem like a godsend for seasonal allergy sufferers, Japanese research confirms that propolis acts like a natural antihistamine.

And Iranian researchers conducted a human trial that showed daily administration of propolis greatly improved long-term asthma symptoms.

Quercetin, a flavonoid found in many fruits and vegetables and in propolis, is largely credited with the anti-inflammatory and immunomodulatory effects that make it so effective against allergies and asthma.

Wound and burn healing: Some of the same findings apply to propolis and its benefits for wound healing, but there is an additional advantage: Propolis has been confirmed to boost collagen production, helping grow new skin cells to replace damaged ones.

Italian researchers credit bee glue with a plethora of wound healing properties:

"Propolis is believed to have antiseptic, antibacterial, antimycotic, astringent, spasmolytic, anti-inflammatory, anesthetic, antioxidant, antifungal, antiulcer, anticancer and immunomodulatory effect," they wrote in their study published in 2015 in the journal, *Burns and Trauma*. The authors suggest that propolis' wound healing effects may be especially important for people with diabetes, who often experience slow wound healing.

Tooth decay: Calcium phosphate is a primary ingredient of dental plaque that causes tooth decay. Propolis has a unique ability to neutralize calcium phosphate, but those same Italian researchers have confirmed that its antibacterial action has been shown to eliminate bacteria in the saliva of people with the serious gum infections, periodontitis and gingivitis.

Acne: Acne is primarily caused by overproduction of oil, the accumulation of dead skin cells that clog pores and the growth of acne-causing bacteria, including staphylococcus strains. It stands to reason that the antibacterial effects of propolis help neutralize those bacteria, but there's more.

Egyptian researchers credit not only the antibacterial effects of propolis, but also its anti-inflammatory and antioxidant effects of propolis with its "highly significant" effectiveness in treating acne.

Gastrointestinal Distress: Humans are susceptible to a wide variety of gastrointestinal woes. Giardia, a parasite most often found in fecal (poop) contamination of food and water resulting in abdominal pain, diarrhea, bloating.

In a Brazilian human study, children and adults with giardiasis, caused by the *Giardia duodenlis trophozoites* parasite, were given propolis. They showed an impressive cure rate between 52% and 60%, whereas those given the conventional drug treatment showed a 40% cure rate.

Propolis is also documented as a safe and effective treatment for gastric ulcers cause by the *H. pylori* bacteria.

At the beginning of this chapter, I noted how impressed I am with the healing powers of propolis. With the information I've given you here, I am sure you are impressed, too.

WHAT YOU NEED TO KNOW

Propolis has formidable and well-documented healing components for a wide variety of health challenges, including:

- Diabetes
- Cold sores
- Genital herpes
- Allergies
- Wound healing
- Tooth decay
- Acne
- Parasites
- Ulcers

CHAPTER 8

What You Need to Know

The profound healing power of propolis is unquestionable. Its value to humans is incontrovertible. Yes, we all need it at one time or another and in these perilous times, we want it.

This product of our bee friends is truly a gift. And with gifts come responsibility. If bees have insufficient bee glue to weatherproof their hives, they will not survive the winter. If a broad variety of bee-killing pathogens enter the hive, it will not survive.

So it is our responsibility, as human consumers of propolis, to ensure that the hives survive and thrive.

That's why you should be looking for a propolis product that is sustainably harvested and processed so that bees and humans alike are winners.

How to find the right propolis product

The first and easiest answer is to look for a product with the label "Committed to Bee Friendly Practices." That will set you on the right path.

I'm sure it goes without saying that you should be looking for a clean product. That may not be as easy as it seems.

Found raw in the hive, propolis is often mixed with wax (which doesn't break down in the body or provide any benefits), dirt, bee's wings and other debris, so a supplemental form that is a clean powder source of plant flavonoids is definitely best.

Additionally, the best extracts will be from sources with a more "controlled" environment—that is, from hives that are well managed so both bees and humans benefit from the exchange. After all, bees need propolis, too, so gathering this precious resource must be done with them in mind as well.

Propolis is a powerful, natural medicine. It is safe and effective, and truly represents an example of humans and nature working together to create the best result—a strong immune defense and optimal good health.

Another aspect of cleanliness in a product is important: It makes me sad to think about it, but there are products on the market that are contaminated with pesticides, antibiotics, heavy metals and more.

How much do you need?

I recommend the following dosages:

- Adults: 200–400 mg propolis daily as a preventive
- Children ages 4 and over: 100 mg propolis daily as a preventive
- Up to 800 mg propolis daily for active infections and viruses

It's safe and effective for adults and children and is especially effective in combatting viruses like the flu, and yes, even the virus that causes COVID 19 as well as a vast range of bacterial, fungal and other microbial infections.

I've said it before, but this thought bears repeating: If you are feeling ill, it's not necessary to define the cause of your illness because, unlike antibiotics or antivirals that only target specific infections, propolis can combat them all.

NOTE: There have been rare allergic reactions to propolis, mostly characterized by skin irritation that disappears as soon as you stop taking it.

CHAPTER 9

Doc to Doc

TO MY READERS: Please feel free to copy this chapter and the reference section of this book and give them to your health care provider. It may be a lifesaver.

Dear Health Care Professional,

Like most books, this book, *Propolis: Nature's Strongest Infection Fighter* by Terry Lemerond, is copyrighted. However, the information presented here is so important to your patients' health and to your scientific knowledge that we have urged our readers to copy this chapter and the reference section and give them to you in hope that this brief summary of efficacy of bee propolis will help you recognize its effectiveness in immune system enhancement and in prevention and treatment of a broad range of disease conditions.

First, let me briefly introduce myself:

I am Alexander Panossian, Ph.D. and Dr.Sci. in bioorganic chemistry, the chemistry of natural and physiologically active compounds. I have been a professor in this discipline since 1991, working in Sweden since 2003 at the Swedish Herbal Institute and as a founder of Phytomed AB in Sweden. I was editor-in-chief of Phytomedicine, an international journal of phytotherapy and phytopharmacology from 2014–2017. I have been credited as lead researcher or participant in more than 180 articles published in peer-reviewed journals, and I hold four US patents. My major interest is in natural botanicals and related medicinals.

From this background, I can enthusiastically support the use of bee propolis as safe and scientifically validated against a broad range of pathogens, including viral, bacterial, fungal and protozoan infections.

If you are unfamiliar with propolis, it is a resin produced by bees to protect their colonies. Not only is "bee glue" used to weatherproof their hives and to quite literally mummify intruders too large for bees to remove before they putrify, it sanitizes and protects the hive from all types of disease.

It has been tested and found efficacious against a wide range of viruses, including the SARS-CoV-2.

Propolis is a powerful antimicrobial with extraordinary value to you and your patients.

To further demonstrate the broad range of efficacy for propolis, it has also been found to be particularly effective against otitis media, dental caries and other oral infections and vaginitis. It is safe for children.

Because of the impressive antimicrobial properties of propolis, "bee glue" can treat a wide range of infections without the need for extensive laboratory work to determine the cause of the infection.

Propolis' broad treatment possibilities

Here is a partial list of conditions where propolis has been validated to prevent, ameliorate or eliminate symptoms:

- Covid-19
- Colds and flu
- Several types of cancer
- HIV
- HPV
- Ebola
- Ulcers
- Cold sores and genital herpes
- Burns and wound healing
- Periodontal disease
- Tooth decay
- Vaginitis
- Acne

And against the following microbes and more:

- *SARS-CoV-2*
- *Staphylococcus aureus*
- *E. coli*
- *Staphylococcus Saprophyticus, Enterococcus Faecalis and Mycobacterium tuberculosis*
- *H1N1, H0N1 and H3N2 viruses*
- *Giardia*
- *Herpes simplex*
- *H. pylori*

Propolis has also been studied and found effective against the following:

Gram-positive bacteria

Bacillus cereus, Bacillus mesentericus, Corynebacterium spp., Corynebacterium diphtheriae, Diplococcus pneumonae, Enterococcus spp., Mycobacteria sp., Mycobacterium tuberculosis, Staphylococcus aureus, Streptococcus: critecus epidermis faecalis mutans, pyogenes, viridans, sobrinus, Micrococcus luteus

Gram-negative bacteria

Branhamella catarrhalis, E. coli, Helicobacter pylori, Klebsiella ozaemae, Klesbsiella pneumonae, Proteus vulgaris, Pseudomonas aeruginosa, Salmonella: choleraesuis, dublin, enteritidis, exneri, gallinarum, pullorum, typhimurium, paratyphi-A, paratyphi-B, typhi Shigella: dysenteriae, sonnei

Antibiotic resistance

I'm sure by now you are beginning to recognize the therapeutic and prophylactic value of propolis for your patients.

There's one other "selling point" vital in today's world: It is a viable alternative treatment for antibiotic resistant infections.

You are undoubtedly aware of the increasing challenges of antibiotic resistance to the greater challenge of finding viable treatments. Propolis offers effective treatment that circumvents antibiotic resistance and has no documented serious side effects.

Cancer

Propolis has also been confirmed efficacious against various forms of cancer, including breast, lung and bronchial, prostate, colorectal, melanoma and several more of the most common and most deadly cancers.

It has been lab, animal and clinically tested with the following results:

- An antioxidant of superior strength
- Anti-angiogenic
- Apoptosis inducing

- Immune system enhancement, primarily through a variety of polyphenols, especially CAPE (caffeic acid phenethyl ester)
- Tumor suppressant
- Antimetastatic
- Chemo enhancement

How to find the right product

I recommend a product based on homogenized propolis harvested from hives in countries surrounding the 45th parallel to assure a broad range of tree resins from which the bees create propolis.

It's important to find a product that is cleanly and sustainably harvested.

I recommend 200–400 mg daily prophylactically and additional doses of up to 800 mg daily for those with active infections or cancer.

—Alexander Panossian, Ph.D., Dr.Sci.

References

Chapter 1: Meet the Beehive's Immune System

Wagh VD. Propolis: A Wonder Bees Product and Its Pharmacological Potentials. *Adv Pharmacol Sci* 2013; 2013: 308249.

Chapter 2: What Bee Glue Means for Humans

Paspuleti VR, Sammugam L, Ramesh N et al. Honey, Propolis, and Royal Jelly: A Comprehensive Review of Their Biological Actions and Health Benefits. *Oxid Med Cell Longev* 2017; 2016: 1259510.

Chapter 3: Vanquish All Kinds of Viruses

Berretta AA, Silveira MA, Capcha JM et al. Propolis against SARS-CoV-2 infection and Covid-19. *Biomed & Pharmaco* Vol 131: 2020 Nov;131: 110622.

Ripari N, Sartori AA, Honorio MS et al. Propolis antiviral and immunomodulatory activity: a review and perspectives for Covid-19 treatment. *J Pharm Pharmacol.* 2021 Feb 8 : rgaa067.

Silviera MD, De Jong D, Berretta AA et al. Efficacy of Brazilian green propolis (EPP-AF®) as an adjunct treatment for hospitalized Covid-19 patients: A randomized, controlled clinical trial. *Biomed Pharmacother.* 2021 Jun;138:111526.

Ali AM, Kunugi H. Propolis, Bee Honey, and Their Components Protect against Coronavirus Disease 2019 (Covid-19): A Review of In Silico, In Vitro, and Clinical Studies. *Molecules* 2021 Feb 25;26(5):1232.

Bachevski D, Damevska K, Simeonovski V et al. Back to the basics: Propolis and Covid-19. *Dermatol Ther.* 2020 Jul;33(4):e13780.

Refaat H,Mady FM, Sarhan HA et al. Optimization and evaluation of propolis liposomes as a promising therapeutic approach for Covid-19. *Int J Pharm.* 2021 Jan 5;592:120028.

Keflie TS, Bielsalski HK. Micronutrients and bioactive substances: Their potential roles in combating Covid-19. *Nutrition.* 2021 Apr;84:111103.

Maruta H, He H. PAK1-blockers: Potential Therapeutics against Covid-19. *Med Drug Discov.* 2020 Jun;6:100039.

Ripari N, Sartori AA, Honorio MS et al. Propolis antiviral and immunomodulatory activity: a review and perspectives for Covid-19 treatment. *J Pharm Pharmacol.* 2021 Mar 6;73(3):281–299.

Chapter 4: Banish Bacteria, Too

Wagh VD. Propolis: A Wonder Bees Product and Its Pharmacological Potentials. *Adv Pharmacol Sci.* 2013; 2013: 308249.

Almuhayawi MS. Review: Propolis as a novel antibacterial agent. *Saudi Journal of Biological Sciences.* 27: 2020 Nov;27(11):3079–3086.

Przybyłek I, Karpiński T. Antibacterial Properties of Propolis. *Molecules.* 2018 Apr; 23(4): 795.

El-Guendouz S, Aazza S, Lyoussi B et al. Moroccan Propolis: A Natural Antioxidant, Antibacterial, and Antibiofilm against *Staphylococcus aureus* with No Induction of Resistance after Continuous Exposure. *Evidence-Based Complementary and Alternative Medicine*, vol. 2018, Article ID 9759240, 19 pages, 2018.

Bryan J, Redden P, Traba C. The mechanism of action of Russian propolis ethanol extracts against two antibiotic-resistant biofilm-forming bacteria. *Lett Appl Microbiol.* 2016 Feb;62(2):192–198.

Chapter 5: Eject All Those Other Nasty, Stubborn Bugs

Koc AN, Silicio S, Kasap F et al. Antifungal activity of the honeybee products against Candida spp. and Trichosporon spp. *J Med Food*. Jan-Feb 2011;14(1-2):128–134.

Capoco IR, Bonfim-Mendonca, Arita GS et al. Propolis Is an Efficient Fungicide and Inhibitor of Biofilm Production by Vaginal Candida albicans. *Evid Based Complement Alternat Med*. 2015; 2015: 287693.

Afrouzan H, Zakeri S, Mehrizi AA. Anti-Plasmodial Assessment of Four Different Iranian Propolis Extracts. *Arch Iran Med*. 2017 May;20(5):270–281.

Chapter 6: Promote Healthy Cells and Shut Out the Bad Ones

Premratanachai P, Chanschao C. Review of the anticancer activities of bee products. *Asian Pac J Trop Biomed*. 2014 May; 4(5): 337–344.

Misir S, Aliyazicioglu Y, Demir S et al. Effect of Turkish Propolis on miRNA Expression, Cell Cycle, and Apoptosis in Human Breast Cancer (MCF-7) Cells. *Nutrition and Cancer*. Volume 72: 2020;72(1):133-145.

Syamsudin PS, Djamil R, Heffen W et al. Apoptosis of human Breast Cancer Cells induced by Ethylacetate Extracts of Propolis. *American Journal of Biochemistry and Biotechnology* 6 (2): 84–88.

Chapter 7: And There's More...

da Silva LM, de Souza P, Al Jaouni SK. Propolis and Its Potential to Treat Gastrointestinal Disorders. *Evid Based Complement Alternat Med*. 2018; 2018: 2035820.

Pasupuleti VR, Sammugam L, Ramesh N et al. Honey, Propolis, and Royal Jelly: A Comprehensive Review of Their Biological Actions and Health Benefits. *Oxid Med Cell Longhev*. 2017; 2017: 1259510.

Martinotti S, Ranzato E. Propolis: a new frontier for wound healing? *Burns and Trauma*: Volume 3, Article number: 9: 2015 Jul 22;3:9.

Zakerish M, Hjenabi LMK, Zaemzadeh N et al. The Effect of Iranian Propolis on Glucose Metabolism, Lipid Profile, Insulin Resistance, Renal Function and Inflammatory Biomarkers in Patients with Type 2 Diabetes Mellitus: A Randomized Double-Blind Clinical Trial. *Sci Rep*. 2019 May 13;9(1):7289.

Hallajzadeh J, Milajeredi, Amirani E et al. Effects of propolis supplementation on glycemic status, lipid profiles, inflammation and oxidative stress, liver enzymes, and body weight: a systematic review and meta-analysis of randomized controlled clinical trials. *J Diabetes Metab Disord*. 2021 Jan 7;20(1):831–843.

Index

acne, 9, 38, 39, 45
aging, 4, 28
allergies, 8, 9, 36–37, 39, 42
angiogenesis, 30–31, 46
antibacterials, 4, 9, 15–21, 37–38
antibiotic resistance, 16–19, 21, 23, 46
antibiotics, 7, 15, 16–19, 21, 23, 46
antibodies, 13, 14
antifungals, 4, 5, 23–24
anti-inflammatories, 4, 13, 16, 38
antimicrobials, 5, 6, 8, 44
antioxidants, 4, 27–28, 38, 46
antiparasitics, 8, 9, 24, 25, 38, 39
antivirals, 4, 9, 10–14, 36
apoptosis, 28–30, 34, 46
artepillin C, 16, 31

bacteria, 4, 5, 8, 9, 15–21, 23, 37, 38, 45–46
   gram-negative, 20, 45
   gram-positive, 20, 45
bee glue. *See* propolis
beehives, 2–3, 4, 5, 6, 7, 10, 15, 21, 40–41, 44, 47

bees. *See* honeybees
blood sugar, 35–36
blood vessels, 30–31
burns, 8, 37, 45

caffeic acid phenethyl ester, 4, 30, 31, 47
calcium phosphate, 37
cancers, 9, 26–34, 45, 46–47
candida, 23–24
Candida albicans, 23
CAPE. *See* caffeic acid phenethyl ester
cells, 4, 27–33, 34, 36, 37, 38
Chaga's disease, 24, 25
chemotherapy, 33, 34, 47
cholesterol, 36
cold sores, 12, 36, 39, 45
colds, 12, 14, 45
collagen, 37
coronaviruses, 10, 12
Covid-19, 10, 12–13, 45
cytokine storms, 12–13

dental plaque, 37
diabetes, 35–36, 37, 39

53

E. coli, 15, 20, 45
ear infections, 22–23, 44
Ebola, 45
ecosystem, 1–2
eosinophils, 36
Eustachian tube, 22–23

farming, 18
flavonoids, 4, 6, 16, 28, 37, 41
Fleming, Alexander, 17
flu. *See* influenza
fluconazole, 3
food crops, 1–2
free radicals, 27–28, 34
fungi, 4, 5, 23–24, 25

galangin, 31
gastrointestinal distress, 23, 25, 38
giardia, 24, 25, 38, 45
giardiasis, 38
gingivitis, 37
glioblastoma, 31
glycosylated hemoglobin (HbA1C), 35–36

H. pylori, 8, 38, 45
H0N1 virus, 12, 45
H1N1 virus, 12, 45
H3N2 virus, 12, 45
herpes, 14, 36, 45
    genital, 36, 39
    oral, 12, 36, 39, 45
herpes simplex virus 1. *See* HSV-1
herpes simplex virus 2. *See* HSV-2
herpes zoster virus, 36
HIV, 12, 14, 45
honey, 2–3
honeybees, 1–4, 5, 6, 7, 10, 11, 15, 40–41, 44
hospitals, 15, 19
HPV, 14, 45
HSV-1, 12, 36, 45
HSV-2, 36, 45
human papillomavirus. *See* HPV
hydroxycinnamic acids, 6
hygiene, 19

immune system, 2–4, 11–12, 13, 14, 16, 23, 27, 30, 34, 36, 43, 47
immunomodulators, 12, 13, 35, 37, 41, 44, 46, 47
infections, 3, 7, 8, 9, 10, 16–18, 44, 46
    bacterial, 4, 5, 8, 9, 15–21, 23, 37, 38, 45–46
    combination, 22–23, 44
    fungal, 4, 5, 23–24, 25
    parasitic, 4, 25, 38, 39
    viral, 9, 10–14, 18, 36, 44, 45
inflammation, 4, 12, 13, 14, 30, 36, 37, 38
influenza, 10, 12, 14, 41, 45

kaempferide, 16
kaempferol, 31

leishmaniasis, 24, 25

malaria, 24, 25
melanoma, 31
metastasis, 27, 31–33
microbes, 3, 5, 6, 8, 12, 22, 35, 44, 45
MRSA, 15, 19
mummification, 3, 7, 44
Mycobacterium tuberculosis, 20, 45

otitis media. *See* ear infections
oxidants, 27
oxidation, 4, 28
oxidative stress, 27
oxygen, 27, 30

parasites, 24, 25, 38, 39
penicillin, 17
periodontal disease, 9, 37, 45
pneumonia, 16, 17
pollination, 1–2
polyphenols, 4, 16, 28, 30, 47
propolis, 2–5, 40–42, 44–47
    benefits, 6, 7–9, 10–14, 19–25, 44–47
    cleanliness of, 40–41, 47
    components, 4, 6, 16, 30, 31
    dosages, 41, 47
    history of, 7–9
    immunomodulatory effect, 12, 13
    name variants, 3, 7
    reactions to, 42
    safety of, 13–14, 16, 44
    sustainably-produced, 40, 47

quercetin, 31, 37

retroviruses, 12

SARS-CoV-2, 11, 12, 14, 44, 45
shingles, 36
Staphylococcus aureus, 9, 15, 19, 45

thrush, 24, 25
tooth decay, 9, 37, 39, 44, 45
toxoplasmosis, 24, 25
trichomoniasis, 24, 25
tuberculosis, 20
tumors, 30–34, 47
    See also cancers

ulcers, 8, 38, 39, 45

vaginitis, 9, 24, 25, 44, 45
viruses, 9, 10–14, 18, 36, 44, 45

wound healing, 7, 8, 37, 39, 45

yeast, 23–24

About the Author

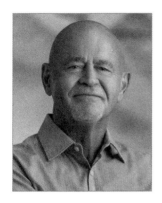

Terry Lemerond is a natural health expert with over 55 years of experience. He has owned health food stores, founded dietary supplement companies, and formulated more than 500 products. A much sought-after speaker and accomplished author, Terry shares his wealth of experience and knowledge in health and nutrition through his educational programs, including the *Terry Talks Nutrition* website (https://www.terrytalksnutrition.com), newsletters, podcasts, webinars, and personal speaking engagements. His books include *Seven Keys to Vibrant Health* and the sequel, *Seven Keys to Unlimited Personal Achievement,* and his newest publication, *50+ Natural Health Secrets Proven to Change Your Life.* His continual dedication, energy, and zeal are part of his on-going mission — to improve the health of America.

KNOWLEDGE IS POWER,
ESPECIALLY FOR YOUR HEALTH!

Are you in search of a reliable, science-based resource for all your health and nutrition questions? Terry Talks Nutrition has you covered.

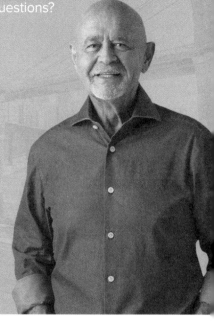

Connect with Terry to increase your knowledge on a wide variety of topics, including immunity, pain, curcumin and cancer, diabetes, and so much more!

READ
Visit TerryTalksNutrition.com for today's latest and greatest health and nutrition information.

LISTEN
Tune in on Sat. and Sun. 8-9 am (CST) at TerryTalksNutrition.com for a live internet radio show hosted by Terry! You can listen to past shows on the website or on your favorite podcast app.

ENGAGE
Connect with us on Facebook, where you can engage with other individuals seeking safe and effective ways to improve overall wellness.

WATCH
Check out our educational YouTube Channel to learn from the world's leading doctors and health experts.

Simply open your smartphone camera. Hold over desired code above for more information.

Get answers to all of your health questions at **TERRYTALKSNUTRITION.COM**

WELCOME TO

ttn publishing

Are you ready to learn how anyone can use natural medicines, safely and effectively, to improve their health? You'll love TTN Publishing, my newest endeavor to bring you cutting edge research on powerful, health-supporting botanicals. I've coauthored numerous books with top alternative doctors from around the world to help you learn all you can about taking your health into your own hands. These educational books, supported by powerful scientific research, contain all the information you need to live a life of vibrant health.

In Good Health,
Terry Lemerond

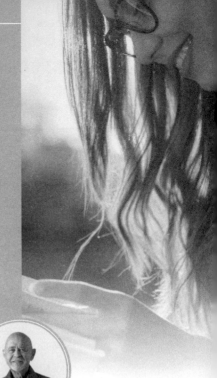

ADDITIONAL BOOKS BY TTN PUBLISHING:

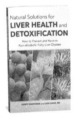 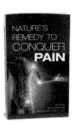 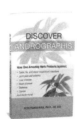 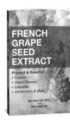 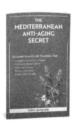 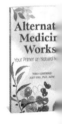

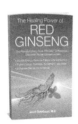 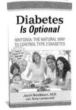 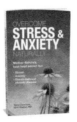 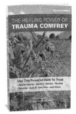 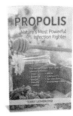 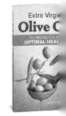

Get a copy for yourself and gift them to the people you care about!

©2024_01_